WHITE

Prescription

ALSO BY CHRISTOPHER VASEY, N.D.

The Acid–Alkaline Diet for Optimum Health
Restore Your Health by Creating pH Balance
in Your Diet

The Detox Mono Diet
The Miracle Grape Cure and Other
Cleansing Diets

The Water Prescription
For Health, Vitality, and Rejuvenation

The
WHEY
Prescription

~

The Healing Miracle in Milk

CHRISTOPHER VASEY, N.D.

TRANSLATED BY JON E. GRAHAM

Healing Arts Press
Rochester, Vermont

Healing Arts Press
One Park Street
Rochester, Vermont 05767
www.HealingArtsPress.com

Healing Arts Press is a division of Inner Traditions International

Originally published in French under the title *La cure de petit-lait: Purifiez votre corps* by Éditions Jouvence, S.A., Chemin du Guillon 20, Case 143, CH-1233 Bernex, Switzerland, www.editions-jouvence.com, info@editions-jouvence.com

First U.S. edition published in 2006 by Healing Arts Press

Note to the reader: This book is intended as an informational guide. The remedies, approaches, and techniques described herein are meant to supplement, and not to be a substitute for, professional medical care or treatment. They should not be used to treat a serious ailment without prior consultation with a qualified health care professional.

Library of Congress Cataloging-in-Publication Data
Vasey, Christopher.
  [Cure de petit-lait. English]
  The whey prescription : the healing miracle in milk / Christopher Vasey ; translated by Jon E. Graham. —1st U.S. ed.
       p. cm.
  Summary: "An introduction to the powerful healing properties of whey" —Provided by publisher.
  Includes bibliographical references and index.
  ISBN-13: 978-1-59477-127-9 (pbk.)
  ISBN-10: 1-59477-127-8 (pbk.)
  1. Whey—Therapeutic use. 2. Milk—Therapeutic use. I. Title.
  RM234.4.V37 2006
  613.2'6—dc22
                                                              2006019661

Printed and bound in Canada by Transcontinental Printing

10 9 8 7 6 5 4 3 2 1

Text design and layout by Jon Desautels
This book was typeset in Sabon with Simplix used as the display typeface

Contents

⤳

May your foods be your medicines.

HIPPOCRATES

1

The History of
Whey

A patient in the city of Zurich, Switzerland, whom the medical treatments of the time were unable to cure and to whom the doctors were giving little time left to live, journeyed to the mountain village of Gais (in the canton of Appenzell Ausserrhoden) in 1749 and was healed of his disease by drinking whey on a daily basis.

Was this patient aware of the past success of treatments based on drinking whey, the liquid known to the Greek doctors of antiquity as "healing water"? Or had he heard the peasants of this mountainous region talk about whey's healing properties?

The History of Whey

⌒

We don't know, but the news soon spread of this patient, who survived despite his doctor's terrible diagnosis, and numerous people with illnesses flooded to Gais to benefit in turn from the miraculous healing properties of whey. A health spa was soon created in this tiny village. It was followed by the opening of more than 160 others in Switzerland, Austria, and Germany. These spas were most active in the middle of the eighteenth century and throughout the nineteenth century. The renowned benefits of the whey cure brought emperors, princes, and aristocrats from all of Europe to take the cure in these spas, to be healed of their ailments or simply to improve their general health.

What is most amazing about whey is that its healing properties have been recognized since antiquity, and modern scientific research has only confirmed the knowledge of the ancients. The whey cure is used today just as it was twenty-four centuries ago. Few remedies or cures can boast of such a long history and such unanimous agreement about their virtues.

Hippocrates (466–377 BCE), the father of medicine, recommended whey to his patients. Following him, Galen (131–200 CE), another founding father of medicine, advised his patients about the whey cure. For a time he even directed a treatment center, sponsored by the famous school of Salerno, at the foot of the "milk mountain" in Italy, between Sorrento and Naples.

Whey cures were also recommended by other famous names from the history of medicine: the Islamic doctor and author of nearly two hundred works, Ibn Sīnā, known in the West as Avicenna (980–1037 CE); Thomas Sydenham (1624–89), the "English Hippocrates," who especially recommended whey for the treatment of gout; Hermann Boerhaave (1668–1738), the famous Dutch physician whose methods of clinical instruction were used throughout Europe; Victor Albrecht von Haller (1708–77), the Swiss biologist, considered the father of neurology, who discovered the function of bile; Christoph Wilhelm Hufeland (1762–1836), the German physician who taught how to prolong life by adopting healthier ways of living; and Samuel Auguste Tissot (1728–97), of Switzerland, remembered for his studies on migraines, which laid the foundation for future research by generations of doctors.

Contrary to what its French name, *petit-lait,* which means "little milk," might suggest, whey is not a poor relative of milk. *While milk is universally esteemed for its nutritional value, whey is valued for its many healing properties.* These properties are enhanced by the fact that whey is easily digested and can be drunk in much larger quantities than milk. Whey's therapeutic activity is beneficial to the major organs of the body: heart, liver, kidneys, and intestines. Its action is cleansing, detoxifying, and regenerative. It has been—and still is—used with success for liver diseases (hepatic insufficiency, hepatitis, gallstones); kidney disorders (infections, kidney stones, edema); intestinal disorders (fermentation, flatulence, constipation, chronic indigestion, bloating); joint diseases (rheumatism, arthritis, osteoarthritis, gout); and against the scourge of modern illnesses, the cardiovascular diseases (high cholesterol, high blood pressure, heart attacks). Whey is also very effective in the fight against excess weight (obesity) and skin disorders (acne, eczema), and for improving general health and well-being.

Like many other remedies, the whey cure has experienced its times of glory and times of oblivion. Those times when the cure was abandoned were not due to the ineffectiveness of whey, but rather to problems involving its preservation—a dilemma that has now been resolved.

Whey is an extremely perishable beverage, which must be consumed within nine to ten hours of its manufacture. Liquid whey quickly spoils, and changes in its taste and odor make it undrinkable. Now, thanks to the fabrication of whey in powder form, its benefits are available to everyone.

The History of Whey

⟿

In the eighteenth- and nineteenth-century health spas, a carefully timed system had to be put in place so that people wishing to take this cure could have whey at their disposal. Whey that had been prepared late at night was carried, at about 3 a.m., from remote mountain cheese makers and after a two- or three-hour walk reached the spa at the first gleams of dawn. The containers that held the whey were carefully wrapped in cloth so that the liquid would hold its heat while being transported and arrive still warm. A ringing bell announced the whey's arrival and it was quickly poured into glasses, each holding about ¼ liter (1 cup), that were lined up on tables for those following the cure. Given the fact that the cure consisted of increasing the quantity consumed each day and, depending on the case, ingesting eight to twelve glasses in a row, new glasses were continually being filled and a bell rang every quarter hour to announce that the time to drink the next glass had arrived.

The whey was still fresh enough in the middle of the morning when the three hours necessary to drink a dozen glasses had elapsed. By the end of the morning the whey was no longer useable, and one would have to wait until the following morning for fresh whey to arrive.

〜

Today, the consumption of reconstituted whey from whey powder makes it easy to follow the cure throughout the day or simply to drink it occasionally for pleasure and general well-being.

2
What Is Whey?

During the manufacture of cheese, milk is curdled by means of rennet. The milk coagulates and a hard part (casein) and a liquid part (whey, also called lactoserum) appear. Whey is therefore the liquid that escapes from the curd when it is left to drain. It is transparent, yellowish-green in color, and possesses a slightly tart flavor that is fairly pleasant.

Whey can also be found in yogurt, which is another form of coagulated milk. The clear liquid that appears on the surface of yogurt when you take out a spoonful is whey. (However, the whey at the top of store-bought yogurt is not fresh and therefore is not beneficial.)

Raw whole cow's milk contains all the nutritional

elements (proteins, vitamins, minerals, and so on) necessary for the growth of the baby calf. When this milk is curdled, these elements will be divided between the casein and the whey. The figures provided in the table below compare the nutrients found in raw milk to the amount of each nutritional element that remains in whey after the casein has been removed.

NUTRITIONAL COMPOSITION PER 100 GRAMS

	Raw Milk	Liquid Whey
Water	87.0 grams	93.3 grams
Carbohydrates	4.7 grams	4.7 grams
Lipids	3.8 grams	0.3 gram
Proteins	3.3 grams	0.9 gram

This table clearly shows the distinctive characteristics of whey. Whey is poor in fats (lipids) and proteins because these two substances primarily remain in the cheese. But it is the exact opposite regarding sugar (carbohydrates): only a negligible amount remains in the cheese and most of it can be found in the whey.

It is important to note that although the protein content of whey is quite small, these proteins are of very high biological value. Furthermore, the sugar that is contained in whey is lactose, a very physiological sugar that the body finds quite easy to metabolize.

When fresh liquid whey is transformed to make powdered whey, the proportion of these different elements changes again. The nutrients are naturally present in higher concentrations in the powdered form because the liquid part has been removed. But with the addition of water, this powder-based whey will reveal a concentration similar to that of fresh whey.

NUTRITIONAL COMPOSITION PER 100 GRAMS

	Liquid Whey	Whey Powder*
Carbohydrates	4.7 grams	75 grams
Lipids	0.3 gram	1 gram
Proteins	0.9 gram	12 grams

*For a more complete analysis see Appendix 2: Nutritional Analysis of Powdered Whey, pages 80–81.

To summarize, whey is a food that is rich in lactose, is practically fat free, and contains proteins of very high biological value. It is quite rich in potassium (but poor in sodium) and contains some of the valuable vitamins found in milk.

Given that the healing virtues of whey depend on the

properties and proportions of the different nutritive substances it contains, we will first take a look at whey's nutritional aspects. We will then look at the basis of its healing properties as well as in what diseases and health disorders its use is indicated. We will end the book with an explanation of how to follow a whey cure.

3

The Nutritional Substances in Whey

LACTOSE

Lactose, also called milk sugar, is the form in which sugar occurs in whey. In fact, lactose is the principal component of whey and is what gives it several of its fundamental properties. In 100 grams of liquid whey there are 4.7 grams of lactose.

As a disaccharide, composed of glucose and galactose, lactose is a sugar that the body finds easy to use; consequently, it is a good energy provider. However, this is only one of its many virtues.

During the digestive process, lactose is not completely

broken down in the stomach at the top of the digestive tract; it is still lactose when it enters the intestines. Far from being any kind of drawback, this is an advantage because the lactose will be transformed into lactic acid by the bacteria of the intestinal flora.

Lactic acid provides numerous benefits to the digestive system. It stimulates intestinal peristalsis—the contractions of the intestinal muscles that push the alimentary bolus (the mass of chewed food) from one end to the other of the long tube of the intestine—thereby guaranteeing a good evacuation of wastes and fecal matters out of the body. Lactic acid acts as a gentle and physiologically appropriate laxative that counteracts intestinal stasis (or laziness) and constipation.

The lactic acid that is produced from the lactose in whey also encourages the assimilation of calcium, phosphorus, potassium, and magnesium, by making these minerals soluble on the intestinal level. "Prepared" in this way by the action of the lactic acid, the minerals are much easier for the intestinal walls to absorb. Once absorbed, they enter the bloodstream, which carries them into the cells where the body can put them to use.

Another vital role played by lactose and lactic acid is the regulation of the intestinal flora, which is achieved by preventing the development of putrefactive bacteria.

The Nutritional Substances in Whey

～

The intestine contains as many bacteria of fermentation as it does bacteria of putrefaction. These two kinds of bacteria are antagonists, because they develop in environments governed by opposing conditions: the bacteria of fermentation in an acid environment, the bacteria of putrefaction in an alkaline environment.

Fermentation and putrefaction are a normal part of the digestive process. However, in certain conditions, one of these two kinds of bacteria will multiply to an excessive extent and the process governed by that bacteria (fermentation or putrefaction) will become pathological.

This takes place when the environment at the end of the small intestine and the beginning of the colon is altered. Here, the environment should be acidic to permit the bacteria of fermentation to perform their task of digesting the cellulose of whole grains, vegetables, and fruits. When a person's diet includes only a small percentage of these foods, the environment will become alkaline instead, thereby encouraging the unbalanced development of putrefying bacteria. These bacteria will then attack the proteins that are passing through this area (from meats, cheeses, and so forth) and cause them to putrefy. Because the intestinal flora is now imbalanced, these will no longer be the normal putrefactions of the digestive process, but pathological putrefactions that produce a large number of toxic substances, including hydrogen sulfide, ammonia, skatole, and indole.

These toxins cause distension, flatulence, and irritation of the intestinal mucous membranes. The damage to the mucous membranes allows the toxins to enter the blood where they cause a latent state of self-poisoning (autointoxication). The severity of gastrointestinal discomfort a person will experience is in direct proportion to the extent of the pathological putrefaction and the quantity of toxins that has resulted.

Whey's contribution of lactose is invaluable because it encourages the rebalancing of the intestinal flora. Lactose is the preferred food of fermenting bacteria; as the environment acidifies with the production of lactic acid, the development of putrefying bacteria is inhibited.

LACTIC ACID

In addition to the lactic acid that is formed from lactose by the action of the bacteria in the intestinal flora, whey already contains lactic acid that was produced by bacteria during the manufacturing of the cheese. In 100 grams of fresh whey, there is approximately 0.5 gram of lactic acid.

Studies have shown that there are two kinds of lactic acid: L+ lactic acid and D- lactic acid. Of these two, L+ is the most beneficial because the body possesses the enzyme that allows the system to make use of it. The lactic acid produced from lactose in the intestines is this more useable form, L+, as is that generated by the muscles as they burn sugars (which in excess can cause muscle aches and stiffness).

The body has greater difficulty using D- lactic acid. Because of its acidic nature and the fact that the body cannot break it down, too large a quantity of the D-type exposes the body to the danger of acidification. The World Health Organization cautions against consuming more than 100 milligrams of D- lactic acid per 2.2 pounds (1 kilogram) of body weight a day. For a person weighing 150 pounds (60 kilos), this amounts to no more than 6000 milligrams, or 6 grams. Infants and children have a reduced capacity to neutralize D lactic acids, so it is even more important that they heed these recommendations.

Now, the lactic acid found in *fresh* whey is entirely L+ lactic acid, the kind that is easily adaptable to human physiology. This is also true for whey in powder form. However, as mentioned earlier, whey is a food that is very hard to preserve. With every passing hour it deteriorates and changes until it becomes undrinkable because the L+ lactic acids are gradually transformed into D- lactic acids. This is why, before the development of the powdered form, whey cures were generally taken in health spas where whey could be consumed immediately after it had been manufactured. The 6-gram daily limit of D- lactic acid can be found in 1.2 liters of *old* whey.

LIPIDS

Whey contains very little fat: 0.3 gram in 100 grams of liquid whey. This is a negligible quantity in principle; in practice, whey is considered to be fat free. This, among other reasons, makes it an ideal food for those dieting to lose weight. (This will be discussed further in the section on weight problems in chapter 5.)

CALORIC INTAKE

There are 26 calories per 100 grams of liquid whey. These calories are not from fats (whey has only a negligible quantity), but from lactose, which as previously mentioned is a sugar that the body can metabolize easily.

Furthermore, the calories provided by whey are full calories rather than the empty calories found in white rice, white sugar, and white bread. Whey calories are accompanied by a number of minerals and vitamins and are therefore much easier for the body to use.

PROTEINS

Whey has very little protein: 0.9 gram per 100 grams of liquid whey (less than 1 percent of its total weight). However, the value of a food's protein contribution is not based only on the quantity of proteins it contains, but also on the body's ability—or lack of ability—to make use of them.

All proteins are not alike; their characteristics depend on the elements of which they are constructed—in other words, the amino acids they contain. There are twenty different amino acids that enter into the composition of *human* proteins. Of these twenty, eight are defined as essential because without each of them, a human protein cannot be constructed. In other words, even if only one of the essential amino acids is missing and all the other amino acids are present in great number, protein construction is impossible.

One essential amino acid cannot be substituted for another and, given the fact that the human body is incapable of manufacturing essential amino acids on its own, it is imperative that they be brought into the body through food. Whey is one of the foods capable of supplying the body with all eight of these essential amino acids. This is one of the reasons for the high biological value of its proteins.

Another reason is the high utilization coefficient of the proteins contained in whey. The human body does not absorb food proteins as they are; it breaks them down in the digestive process into isolated amino acids and then recombines them into human protein. During this process, there are amino acids that cannot be utilized. The body has to break them down even further, and this process produces toxins that the kidneys and skin will have to eliminate. The more amino acids that cannot be used by the system, the lower the coefficient of utilization and the less value the proteins of the food are considered to have.

Knowledge of the utilization coefficient of different proteins is of extreme importance when it comes to supplying a patient with optimum nutrition or to reducing the quantity of protein wastes to be eliminated. Waste reduction is especially important in kidney diseases.

It so happens that the utilization coefficient of whey's proteins is quite high, much higher than that of milk, eggs, or meat. Recent studies have shown that the overall composition of amino acids in whey is identical to that of human blood.

MINERALS

Whey is a food that is especially rich in mineral salts. They amount to 5 percent of its total weight. The principal minerals found in whey will be discussed in this section.

Potassium

Whey is extremely rich in potassium. Potassium plays an essential role in the processes of assimilation and catabolism on the cellular level, in the transmission of nerve impulses, and in muscular contractions (if there is a potassium deficiency, cramps occur). Furthermore, it is an activator of numerous enzymes.

Potassium is also a foe of sodium (salt), which means that the more potassium there is in the tissues the greater the amount of sodium is driven out of the body, and with it the water it retains. Each gram of salt retains 11 grams of water. By driving out the excess sodium, potassium triggers a powerful diuretic effect. In the case of a potassium deficiency, more sodium collects in the tissues and with it excess fluid causing edema (an abnormal accumulation of fluid).

The high amount of potassium in whey provides the foundation for its principal healing virtues: its diuretic action and its ability to eliminate toxins.

Calcium

Whey is a valuable source of calcium, which is an indispensable mineral for building and maintaining strong, healthy bones and teeth and is necessary for the transmission of nerve impulses. Calcium is especially recommended for children and those who are pregnant or nursing because the system's need for calcium is much greater at these time.

Calcium deficiency can lead to diseases such as osteoporosis, hypersensitive nerves, insomnia, and rickets.

Magnesium

Whey also contains magnesium, which has important functions in the nervous system, where it simultaneously strengthens and relaxes, and in the immune system, whose defensive capacities it reinforces. In addition to its antiviral action, magnesium lowers blood cholesterol and inhibits sclerosis in the blood vessels, both of which benefit the entire cardiovascular system by helping the heart perform its duties.

Phosphorus

Phosphorus is a very useful substance for the nervous system and for brain functions. A deficiency in phosphorus will cause mental fatigue, reducing the brain's ability to concentrate and remember. Phosphorus, which is present in whey, is therefore highly recommended in cases of memory loss.

Sodium

Whey is known for having very low sodium. This is particularly important because excess salt in the tissues will retain water, and with this water, toxins, which can cause high blood pressure, tire the heart and overwork the kidneys, which are responsible for eliminating salt from the body.

The fact that whey is rich in potassium, the enemy of salt, and at the same time contains very little sodium itself, reinforces the beneficial aspects of its low-sodium nature.

VITAMINS

In addition to the minerals we just examined, whey also contains vitamins, though in somewhat lesser quantities. Vitamins A, B_1, B_2, B_3, B_5, B_6, C, D, and E are present in whey. Of these, it possesses the greatest quantity of B_2, or riboflavin.

A deficiency of vitamin B_2 will lead to an exaggerated sensitivity of the eyes to light (as does a vitamin A deficiency), a tendency to tearing, red eyes, red blotches on the face, oily and puffy skin, and cracks at the edges of the lips.

The Nutritive Value of Whey

- Rich in lactose
- Contains no fat and is therefore low in calories
- Contains proteins of high biological value
- Rich in minerals (especially potassium)
- Good source of vitamin B_2

4

The Healing
Properties of
Whey

Whey's benefits are not limited to its nutritious properties; it also has numerous healing properties. Contrary to
other remedies or foods that act only on a single organ
or in a single manner, whey's healing action works in
multiple fashions. It acts on the intestines, liver, and kidneys, while encouraging assimilatory and eliminatory
functions. This chapter will detail the multivalent healing properties of whey.

A GENTLE BUT EFFECTIVE
INTESTINAL LAXATIVE

With the lactic acid present in whey, along with the lactic acid produced by the lactose it contains, whey stimulates intestinal peristalsis.

The intestines must evacuate feces in order to avoid becoming poisoned by their own wastes. The matter in the intestines makes its way through them thanks to the contractions of the circular muscles of the intestinal walls. As these contract in successive waves (peristaltic movement), they tighten the available space and push the wastes forward in the direction of the exit out of the body.

The muscles responsible for intestinal peristalsis can be stimulated in two ways. There is the mechanical way: food fiber (wheat bran, oat bran, cellulose contained in fruits and vegetables) fills the intestine, thus reflexively triggering the peristaltic process. Then there is the chemical way, activated by the presence of specific stimulating substances (the active substances of various medicinal plants or, in the case that concerns us specifically, the lactic acid of whey).

Rather than having a purgative effect, whey is a quite gentle laxative. It is effective in the case of intestinal sluggishness as well as for both occasional and chronic constipation. It has even sometimes provided excellent results in cases where the intestines have been exhausted by the overuse of purges and harsh chemical laxatives.

REGENERATING THE INTESTINAL FLORA

The lactose content of whey inhibits the presence of bacteria that causes putrefaction and encourages the functions performed by the beneficial bacteria. By helping the intestinal flora regenerate, whey has a beneficial effect on the digestive process. When intestinal flora is partially destroyed or imbalanced, the transformation of foods is poorly achieved, which can cause a number of chronic digestive disorders. Taking whey regularly can cure these problems and restore normal digestive function. The stools reacquire their normal consistency (neither too hard as is the case with constipation, nor too soft as occurs with diarrhea) and lose their foul odor. Flatulence and bloating also disappear. Lactose is the nourishment of choice for the beneficial bacteria of the intestinal floras, because it allows them to reproduce and multiply much more easily. Because many adults have difficulty digesting milk, whey, which is easily digested, is an ideal source of this lactose. It is therefore particularly useful to consume whey at times when the microorganisms of the intestinal flora have been destroyed, for example when antibiotics have been taken.

STIMULATING AND DETOXIFYING THE LIVER

Whey has an indirect effect on the liver; it works on it by way of the intestines. The liver is quite dependent on the condition of the intestines, because substances are transported from the intestine to the liver by the portal vein. The liver's role is to store the nutrients or release them into the bloodstream; it is also to neutralize, purify, and eliminate toxic substances.

Although the liver has a high neutralizing and detoxifying capacity, a daily intake of toxins from the intestines can exhaust and exceed its abilities over time. This is exactly what happens when the intestines do not eliminate their wastes on a regular basis (constipation) or when putrefaction occurs ceaselessly because an imbalance in the intestinal flora is producing large quantities of poison (indoles and skatoles): two disorders for which whey provides an excellent remedy!

When the liver becomes exhausted, it can no longer neutralize all the toxins that come its way. These toxins will gradually poison the entire system (see more on this in Correcting the Body's Internal Cellular Environment, beginning on page 32). Further, the exhausted liver can no longer secrete enough bile—a digestive juice that is necessary for the intestines to perform their digestive and eliminatory functions. As a result, there will be poor and incomplete digestion; putrefaction will increase, producing numerous poisons that irritate the intestinal walls and create microlesions. The intestinal mucous membranes, instead of acting as filters, will become porous and allow toxins to enter the bloodstream where they will make

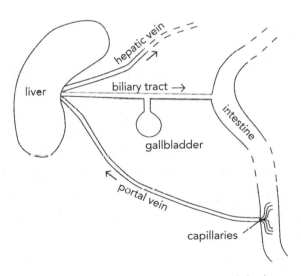

The interdependence of the intestine and the liver

their way to the liver. There—and this quickly turns into a vicious circle—they will exhaust the liver.

Whey has been used effectively to treat hepatic disorders and poisoning since antiquity. Thanks to the whey cure, regeneration and stimulation of the hepatic functions are possible by way of the intestines. Whey, by cleansing the intestinal environment and restoring intestinal flora, encourages good digestion and normal elimination, and this prevents the liver from being assailed by constant waves of toxins. The liver can then detoxify its own tissues and start working normally again, including producing enough bile to ensure good digestion and elimination (bile has a laxative effect).

ELIMINATING EXCESS WATER FROM THE TISSUES

Bodily tissues hold a certain amount of fluids that are retained there by, among other things, the presence of salt. Consequently, there is a physiologically beneficial salt content in the body. In certain pathological situations, however, this content can increase; this naturally results in an increase of the amount of fluid that is held. Edemas will appear, often in the legs (particularly around the ankles), the hands (making it difficult to remove rings), and the eyelids. Because this additional water content has caused the tissues that make up the various organs to swell, numerous health problems can result, including high blood pressure, blood or lymphatic stasis, and organ congestion.

Taking whey, which is rich in potassium, is quite useful in these situations because potassium is the natural enemy of salt and expels it from the body along with the water it has retained. Whey does not create imbalance in the mineral composition of bodily fluids as chemical diuretics can. It expels only excess water the tissues are holding, and not the constituent fluid that is normally present.

A large fluid elimination is one of the more visible and spectacular effects of the whey cure. The quantities of urine that are eliminated are clearly higher than the quantities of water ingested, especially when the individual has been retaining water.

STIMULATING TOXIN ELIMINATION BY THE KIDNEYS

The kidneys are one of the main organs for the elimination of wastes and metabolic residues. They filter wastes out of the blood and eliminate them in a diluted form as urine. The kidneys are constantly working to maintain the composition of the blood as close to its ideal state as possible.

The wastes eliminated by the kidneys include urea, uric acid, creatinine, salts, and expended minerals. For various reasons, however, this elimination can take place in an insufficient manner. Unable to exit the blood, the wastes collect in the body where they can cause various disorders. Gout, for example, is a disease caused by the presence of too much uric acid in the body, acid the kidneys should be eliminating. This disease is displayed by very painful crises of acute arthritis, generally located in the big toe.

Other diseases caused by poor renal elimination include rheumatism, osteoarthritis, and some forms of eczema. The kidneys themselves can also be afflicted when wastes collect in their filters.

During a whey cure, the heightened levels of liquid traveling through the kidneys support the transport and elimination of toxins. This cleans out the renal filter, thereby increasing the possibilities for waste evacuation, and allows the wastes carried to the kidneys by the blood to be much more easily and copiously eliminated. The end result is a general cleansing of the entire system.

Blood analysis after whey cures confirms that the blood has rid itself of numerous wastes. This is also evident by the fact that the symptoms of diseases will diminish in intensity or disappear altogether.

ENCOURAGING ASSIMILATION

Assimilation, by which is meant the cells' potential to receive all the nutritive substances they need (proteins, lipids, carbohydrates, minerals, trace elements, and vitamins), is improved by whey in three different ways.

1. Minerals are transformed into a soluble state by lactic acid, making them easier to assimilate.
2. Whey encourages good digestion (by regenerating intestinal flora), which is essential for nutrients to be extracted from foods and made available for the intestinal mucous membranes to absorb.
3. The restoration of a healthy and clean intestinal environment prevents many of the nutrients that enter the intestines from being destroyed by the poisons caused by putrefaction.

〜

CORRECTING THE BODY'S INTERNAL CELLULAR ENVIRONMENT

All the healing properties of whey discussed in this chapter can be summarized into one general property: *whey provides corrective action to the internal cellular environment.*

The term *internal cellular environment* is used to designate the physical environment in which all the organs of the body reside. Just as the quality of life for human beings depends on their environment (air quality, water quality, food quality, and so forth), the quality of life for our organs (and therefore our entire body) depends on their surroundings, the internal cellular environment. This consists of four bodily fluids: blood, lymph, the fluids that surround the cells (extracellular or interstitial fluid), and the fluids found inside the cells (intracellular fluid). These four fluids alone account for 70 percent of total body weight.

Our organs literally bathe in these fluids and are completely dependent upon them. The fluids eliminate wastes from the organs and bring to them the nutritive substances they need. When the ideal composition of a bodily fluid is altered, the good working order and even the survival of the cells making up the organs are put in danger. For good health, it is imperative that the internal cellular environment maintain its unique properties.

The internal environment can deteriorate, making it easier for disease to appear, in two ways: it can become overloaded with toxins or it can be deficient in the nutritive substances it requires to function.

The principal cause of excess toxins, besides overeating, is insufficient elimination of wastes by the emunctory or excretory organs (the organs responsible for the filtration and elimination of toxins). There are five excretory organs: the liver, intestines, kidneys, skin, and lungs. The liver eliminates wastes through bile, the intestines through fecal matter, the kidneys by urine, the skin by sweat (through the sudoriferous glands) and by sebum (through the sebaceous glands), and the lungs with the air they exhale.

A deficiency in nutritive substances generally originates with intake: either the individual does not eat certain foods or the foods he or she eats do not provide these substances (either because they are naturally deficient or because the nutrients have been lost, as in refined foods). However, another common problem is the deficiency of utilization. In this case, the nutritive substances are brought in by the individual's diet, but they cannot be assimilated and utilized because they are not absorbed or they are destroyed by intestinal poisons.

In naturopathic medicine, the deterioration of the internal cellular environment (caused by deficiencies or an accumulation of toxins) is considered to be the cause of all our health problems. *Illnesses are the visible expression of deep-seated disorders and infections that are welcomed into the body by a deficient cellular environment.*

For example, gout, which we discussed earlier, is not, despite appearances, a disease that is localized in the toes. Gout manifests when the internal cellular environment is overloaded with uric acid. Certainly, the symptoms appear in a particular place on the body (the big toe), but uric acid is saturating the entirety of the system.

The same is true for all diseases: they are never in fact circumscribed to a restricted part of the body, but are the localized expression of a general deterioration of the internal cellular environment.

Therefore, a logical and effective therapy should aim not only to bring about the disappearance of the symptoms of illness, but also to remove its causes by correcting the state of the internal cellular environment. This can be done by dislodging embedded toxins and correcting deficiencies.

Thanks to its multiple healing properties, whey provides invaluable assistance in attaining this double objective. Whey acts on the three main excretory organs:

the liver, the kidneys, and the intestines. It stimulates their eliminatory function, and thus the cleansing of the internal environment. Whey also helps to compensate for deficiencies by the valuable nutrients it contains. In addition, whey encourages the assimilation of these substances by regenerating intestinal flora and aiding digestion.

Over the long term, whey cures can therefore provide an effective contribution to the correction of the body's internal cellular environment.

5

Principal Indications for the Whey Cure

The health concerns that can be affected positively by whey cures will be listed here—ranging from general concerns, such as fatigue and the effects of antibiotic treatment, to serious ailments such as cardiovascular diseases.

For each, a short explanation of the causes of the disease will be provided along with the manner in which whey can act on the disorders. This is by no means an exhaustive list; as we have seen, thanks to its general action of correcting the body's internal cellular environment, numerous other problems can be cured by whey.

Therefore, only the principal indications will be dealt with here.

ANTIBIOTIC TREATMENT

Digestive problems (indigestion, gas, diarrhea) are possible side effects of antibiotic treatments; antibiotics in fact destroy the beneficial bacteria of the intestinal flora. The lactose contained in whey allows this intestinal flora to rebuild itself more quickly and easily.

ATHLETIC ACTIVITIES

When the muscles are worked, acid wastes are produced that reduce the body's resistance and strength. By encouraging elimination of acid through the kidneys, whey allows athletes to increase the time they are able to perform or work out; it also reduces the time necessary for recuperation afterward.

BLADDER INFECTIONS

Certain forms of cystitis (bladder infection) occur when the intestinal flora is out of balance and its microorganisms mutate and become virulent. Whey acts directly on the intestinal flora, working to correct the imbalance while also expelling microbes from the bladder by diuresis.

BLOOD VISCOSITY AND HIGH CHOLESTEROL

Blood is the principal link in the chain of cardiovascular disorders. The wastes transported by blood become deposited on the walls of the vessels and the walls of the heart, hindering blood flow and blocking its passage to a greater extent as time goes by. The purifying action of whey on the liver, kidneys, and intestines helps blood retain its purity and fluidity.

CONSTIPATION OR INTESTINAL LAZINESS

When an intestine is described as lazy, it means that it empties itself only on an episodic basis and does not evacuate all its contents; this occurs when intestinal peristalsis is insufficient. Peristalsis can be stimulated by the lactic acid and lactose that whey brings into the body. Whey has even proven effective at reeducating intestinal function among those people who have relied too heavily on the use of laxatives and purgatives to do what their bodies could no longer do.

DIABETES

Whey helps reduce sugar levels in the blood by stimulating the work performed by the liver and kidneys. Its lactose is suitable for consumption by diabetics, but the amount ingested must be calculated. Three level tablespoons of powdered whey are equal to one serving of bread.

FATIGUE, LACK OF ENERGY AND ENTHUSIASM

When it is not a result of overwork, lack of sleep, or stress, fatigue is often due to the fact that the body cannot function freely because of the toxins that are clogging the system. By cleansing the body, whey contributes to the restoration of normal energy circulation.

GAS AND BLOATING

Because whey supports and restores the beneficial bacteria of the intestinal flora, it prevents putrefaction and the production of gas.

HEART ATTACK AND STROKE

After the emergency treatment required, whey makes it possible to correct the internal environment that is ultimately the cause of the disorders (blood viscosity, excess weight, high blood pressure).

HEMORRHOIDS

Hemorrhoids are varicose veins in the anus with four possible causes: local irritations from intestinal toxins, deformation of the vessel resulting from excessive pressure by fecal matter, liver congestion, and high viscosity of the blood. The properties of whey will act on all four of these causes and therefore provide effective treatment for hemorrhoids.

HIGH BLOOD PRESSURE

There are numerous causes of high blood pressure. Whey acts effectively upon the following: excessive viscosity of the blood, water retention, excess salt in the tissues, and even clogging of the vessels and kidneys.

INDIGESTION

The lactose provided by whey is the food of choice for intestinal flora, which plays an important role in the digestive process. Whey also allows for better digestion through the support it offers the liver by encouraging the production of bile, a digestive fluid that is essential for the digestion of fatty substances. Whey is therefore an ideal treatment for chronic indigestion.

JOINT DISEASES

Rheumatic disorders, such as arthritis, osteoarthritis, gout, and sciatica, are caused by toxins that attack and create lesions in the joints, toxins deposited in the interspatial area of the joints, and the demineralization of the cartilage and bone by acids. The chronic nature of these problems stems from poor diet and poor elimination. The detoxifying and mineral-restoring properties of whey therefore contribute valuable assistance to the treatment of all these diseases.

KIDNEY DISEASES

Whey is a physiologically suitable diuretic that will not irritate diseased kidneys.

KIDNEY STONES

When the kidneys are working too slowly, wastes will collect in their tissues and tubular areas in the form of grit or stones. The diuretic effect of whey stimulates the kidneys and increases the amount of fluid that is transiting through them, thereby ridding the kidneys of these deposits.

LIVER DISEASES AND INSUFFICIENCIES

By cleansing the intestinal environment, whey provides relief to the liver, which can then regenerate and begin functioning more actively again. Whey can be used in cases of hepatic laziness, gallstones, jaundice, and cirrhosis.

MUSCULAR SPASMS AND CRAMPS

Muscular spasms and cramps are often due to deficiencies in potassium and magnesium and are easily remedied by the high content of potassium and other minerals in whey.

SKIN DISORDERS

The skin is the mirror of the body, reflecting the state of the internal cellular environment. When the main excretory organs are not sufficiently ridding the body of its wastes and the body becomes overloaded with toxins, it will seek to eliminate them through the skin. If the presence of toxins is too large, they will congest the sudoriferous and sebaceous glands and irritate the skin, causing pimples and producing eczema and other skin disorders.

The treatment of skin disorders, therefore, should be targeted less at the surface level of the skin; it should involve detoxification of the entire body and rebalancing of the intestinal environment, which is the primary source of wastes.

WATER RETENTION AND EDEMA

Because of its high potassium content and the diuretic effect that potassium has on the system, whey effectively expels excess water being retained in the body.

WEIGHT PROBLEMS

Whey is an ideal food for a weight-loss diet. It helps the body rid itself of wastes and excess water. As natural as bread and potatoes, whey can be eaten on a daily basis. Although it is dietetic, it still provides a small protein base, a light energy boost, and numerous minerals that permit the body to continue performing necessary tasks. Furthermore, eaten half an hour before meals, whey will reduce the sensation of hunger.

6

The Practice of
the Cure

WHAT KIND OF WHEY
SHOULD I USE?

The whey cure can be followed using fresh liquid whey, as our ancestors did in the past, or whey reconstituted from powder.

Fresh Liquid Whey

Whey, in its natural liquid form, will go bad fairly quickly, so fresh whey should be used only by those who can obtain it directly from a cheese maker. Fresh whey should be drunk at once in the two to three hours after its manufacture.

Powdered Whey

If fresh whey is not available, the cure can be taken with whey prepared from powder. The manufacturing methods carefully preserve the properties of the whey almost in their totality. With cold or lukewarm water added to the powdered whey, a drink of whey can be reconstituted instantaneously. To obtain a concentration that is comparable to that of fresh whey, follow the instructions supplied by the product manufacturer. Different brands of whey powders are available commercially.

A company called Biosana makes natural fruit-based powdered whey and supplemental whey tablets, both of which are available in many different flavors (including raspberry, lemon, apple, vanilla, chocolate, and mocha). The possibility this offers for flavor variation is not a negligible consideration during cures of long duration. (See the resources section on page 82 for further information on whey manufacturers and distributors.)

Note: Whey will turn bad quickly whether fresh or prepared from powder. Make sure to prepare each glass of whey when needed; do not make a batch of it at the beginning of the day to be consumed later.

~

DOSAGE

The dosages provided for the whey cure are based on an average. As with any cure, because of the wide variety of individual reactions and physical sensitivities of the people taking the cure—their specific diseases or disorders, age, and vitality—dosage should be determined on a case-by-case basis. It should be reduced if the effects of the cure are too violent and increased when necessary (that is, if the body is not eliminating enough wastes).

THE WHEY CURE

On the first day of the cure, drink ¼ liter (1 cup) of whey. Every day thenceforward, add another ¼-liter dose until the ultimate desired amount has been reached. As previously discussed, dosage will vary depending on the specific case. For most people, the final amount to work up to should be between 2 and 3 liters. The ¼-liter doses should be drunk every fifteen minutes.

When the maximum amount has been reached, gradually reduce the dosage by ¼-liter increments per day until back to the original amount of ¼ liter. This means that, depending on the ultimate amount chosen, the cure will last anywhere from six to twenty-four days.

For people who cannot tolerate drinking large quantities of liquid at one time and begin to feel sick with too much water in their stomachs, it is possible to set a length of twenty-one days to the cure, during which the amount of whey drunk every day will not change, for example 1 liter (or a little more than a quart) a day. The whey should still be drunk in ¼-liter doses every fifteen minutes until the desired amount has been consumed.

Whey should be drunk first thing in the morning. Breakfast, if it is eaten, should be very light. It is best to skip breakfast entirely (consuming only whey) and eat your first meal of the day at noon.

Whey Cure Variation

Instead of concentrating the ingestion of whey over a short span of time—two or three hours in the morning, as with the original cure—this variation allows the whey to be consumed over the course of the entire day. The ¼-liter ration is drunk once an hour instead of every fifteen minutes. In this cure, too, the dosage is increased by ¼ liter a day until the maximum quantity desired has been obtained; then reduced on the same gradual basis. For those who prefer, the duration between doses of whey can be spaced out to an even greater extent among four set times: at rising, at the end of the morn-

ing, at the end of the afternoon, and just before going
to bed.

THE WHEY CURE AND DIET

The beneficial effects of the whey cure will be obvious
even if one does no more than take the whey. However, these effects can be reinforced when the whey cure
is followed in conjunction with a restrictive diet. Any
restriction of food intake will trigger additional healing
phenomena in the body; the greater the restriction, the
more powerful the healing will be.

The first of these healing phenomena is the autolysis
of wastes and diseased tissues. The word *autolysis* literally means digestion (lysis) of one's self (auto). Because
food is restricted, the body no longer receives all the
nutrients it needs, so it draws these substances from its
own tissues. This autolysis does not occur in a random
manner: the first things to be self-digested are wastes and
diseased tissues.

The second healing phenomenon that is set in motion
by dieting is a kind of eliminatory system overhaul and
updating. Because the food intake has been reduced, the
digestive system has less work to perform. The energy
that is saved can be used for eliminatory functions: the

liver, the kidneys, and the intestines all work much more actively to eliminate toxins.*

Following a restrictive diet while taking the whey cure increases its beneficial effects. Three different levels of restriction are outlined in this section; each can be applied to the whey cure with any of the dosage schedules previously discussed.

General Version

Normal food intake is maintained, with the only difference being the addition of whey to the diet. This is the simplest version of the cure.

Strict Version

All foods are removed from the diet and only whey is consumed. This is a mono diet, which means a diet in which only one food is eaten exclusively. There are many different kinds of mono diets—the grape mono diet, the rice mono diet, the carrot mono diet, and so forth—and this would simply be a whey mono diet.

This is the most intensive version of the cure, in which the healing phenomena will take place with the most potency. This variation should not be followed

---

*For more on autolysis and eliminatory updating, see my book *The Detox Mono Diet* (Rochester, Vt.: Healing Arts Press, 2006).

unless you are already very familiar with the practice of mono diets or are under the supervision of a competent health care professional.

Intermediate Version

This variation sits halfway between the general version and the strict version. The intake of food is reduced in order to take advantage of the phenomena of autolysis and eliminatory updating that naturally occur with any diet; but the restriction is not as great as it is in the mono diet, so the cure is easier to tolerate. The diet can be restricted to varying degrees, so it is easily adaptable to the tastes and preferences of the individual.

The restriction can be quantitative: reducing daily food intake by one quarter or one half of the amount of food normally eaten in a day (measured in either grams or calories). For example, instead of eating 3200 calories, allow yourself no more than 2400 or even 1600 calories a day.

The restriction can also be qualitative: in this case the restriction would be based on certain foods, such as meats, animal products, and other foods that are difficult to digest. For example, you could eat what you generally eat, excluding meat and fish (a vegetarian diet). Or, you could omit from your normal diet all meat, fish, and any other kind of animal products, such as cheese and eggs (a vegan diet). To make the diet even more intensive, omit all cereal grains and flours in addition to all animal products. This would result in a diet consisting of only fruits and vegetables, eaten as desired: cooked (by themselves or in vegetable broth), raw, or juiced.

CONTRAINDICATIONS

There is only one contraindication for the whey cure: lactose intolerance. This intolerance manifests by acidic diarrhea and lactosuria (elimination of lactose through the urine). Those who are lactose intolerant are fully aware of their condition, so they will know ahead of time that they should not follow the whey cure.

7

Supplementing the Whey Cure

Adding complementary treatments to the whey cure helps to ensure that the elimination of toxins will be carried through properly. The whey cure causes wastes to emerge from deep within the tissues. This means that there will be an increased amount of toxins rising from the depths of the system and appearing at the various excretory organs to be filtered and eliminated by means of urine, stools, and sweat. It is therefore extremely important that these wastes be able to exit the body, which is possible only if the excretory organs are functioning sufficiently.

Very often, if someone has accumulated toxins and feels the need to get rid of them through a detoxifying cure, it is because the excretory organs have been unable to meet the demands made upon them by the individual's normal intake and production of wastes. Will the cure suddenly give these organs the ability to meet these demands that much better?

The properties of whey *will* specifically stimulate the body's eliminatory organs to work. But because the mass of wastes that need to be eliminated is much larger than usual, the organs may not be able to keep up. Using medicinal plants and increasing physical exercise are two of the supplemental techniques discussed in this chapter that can help maintain and stimulate the labor of the excretory organs.

As wastes are released in greater quantities, the cure will engender various minor disorders known as healing crises, including headaches, fatigue, eczema, pimples, and even the temporary resurgence of former health problems. These healing crises are the normal consequence of the increase in circulating toxins, and their intensity and duration are directly proportionate to how well or how poorly the excretory organs are functioning. By supporting the work of elimination with supplemental treatments, one can avoid overly violent healing crises and also be assured that the wastes are not merely changing location in the body but are genuinely clearing out.

MEDICINAL PLANTS

The health benefits of the whey cure come from the cleansing of the body that is achieved by whey's stimulation of the system to eliminate wastes and toxins. For this reason, it has been common practice throughout history to use depurative (purifying) plants and herbs to reinforce the effects of the cure.

There are several ways to benefit from the effects of medicinal plants. One method is to pasture the livestock whose milk provides the whey in fields that are rich in these plants; thus, the plants' active principles will be contained in the whey. Another option is to ingest the herbs directly in their many available forms.

There are three plants that are commonly recommended as supplements to the whey cure: dandelions, artichokes, and nettles.

Dandelion stimulates the production and elimination of bile and thereby the filtration of wastes and their evacuation out of the system, because bile is the fluid in which wastes are excreted. Thanks to its hepatic action, dandelion acts as a gentle laxative, guaranteeing good intestinal elimination. Dandelion also activates the kidneys' function of purifying the blood by increasing the volume of urine and wastes eliminated over the course of the day.

Artichoke is excellent for draining the liver and the gallbladder; it is also a fine diuretic. It encourages the elimination of urea, cholesterol, and uric acid. Artichoke facilitates the excretion of toxins from the tissues by encouraging cellular exchanges through its stimulation of the circulatory system.

In addition to its diuretic and hepatic qualities, nettle has a tonic property that stimulates circulation and metabolism. Nettle is often used in treatments for rheumatism, eczema, gallstones, and kidney stones—diseases characterized by an accumulation of wastes.

These three plants, or any other depurative plant you might choose, can be used as infusions, drops, tablets, and juices. While the last three do have the advantage of being practical, they do not lead, as do infusions, to the ingestion of a large volume of water. A large intake of liquid is valuable because it supports the transport of toxins and stimulates diuresis by the pressure it places upon the kidneys.

‿

Dosage amounts for drops, tablets, and juices are provided in the manufacturer's instructions. To make an infusion, add 50 grams of dried leaves (about a handful) for every liter of boiled water. Let the leaves steep for ten to fifteen minutes, strain, and drink over the course of the day. The depurative effect should be quite apparent: the frequency of urination, quantity of urine eliminated, and intestinal transit should all increase markedly. Individual systems will respond differently to the plants, so the dosage should be increased or decreased depending on the effect they produce.

Taking medicinal plants in small doses over the course of the entire day stimulates the excretory organs repeatedly, and this, little by little, creates a new working rhythm for them, one that may well persist after the cure is over.

OXYGENATION

Stimulating the work of the excretory organs with whey and medicinal plants allows large quantities of wastes to be eliminated from the body. However, some wastes lie stagnant in the depths of the tissues for so long that they combine with other wastes to form agglomerations.

Because of their large size, they cannot be eliminated naturally without first being broken down into smaller pieces.

The degradation of large toxins into smaller toxins is performed by oxidation. In the presence of oxygen and thanks to enzymatic activity, the wastes are "burned." This combustion results in a fine ash that the body can easily carry to the excretory organs for elimination.

For oxidation to take place successfully, enough oxygen must penetrate the deep tissues. Respiration, because of the sedentary lives most of us lead, generally brings very little oxygen into the body. Furthermore, this oxygen has a difficult time reaching deeper into the tissues, again because our far-too-sedentary lifestyles do not encourage optimum cellular irrigation or exchange.

Physical activities that cause an intensification of the rate of respiration and the sensation of being out of breath will bring more oxygen into the tissues. Walking at a sustained pace, for example, or over uneven terrain will create this healthy oxygenation. Sports activities in general, as well as dancing and manual labor, such as sawing wood, mowing the lawn, and raking leaves, can also have the same result.

The health spas where the whey cure was followed in the eighteenth and nineteenth centuries were most often located in the country and in mountainous regions; long walks in the fresh air were an integral part of the cure.

PHYSICAL EXERCISE

The principal virtue of physical exercise during the whey cure is that it intensifies cellular exchanges and circulation, thereby triggering the movement of deeply embedded toxins toward the surface where they can be expelled. When muscles contract, they have a crushing effect on the surrounding tissues and organs that pushes out some of the bodily fluids and toxins they contain. The action is similar to squeezing a sponge so that it will release the dirty water it contains. The repetition of these contractions engenders a kind of "agitation" in the tissues, which until this point have been only sluggishly irrigated, and releases numerous toxins into the blood where they will travel to the excretory organs. Our tissues are often so poorly irrigated that descriptions such as "marsh" or "desert" are used in natural medicine to designate those regions of the body where capillary and lymphatic circulation are extremely deficient.

Another benefit of exercise during the cure is, as we saw earlier, to encourage oxygenation of the deep tissues and therefore the combustion of the wastes they contain. This combustion is amplified during exercise by the simple fact that the body's energetic needs are increased and this forces the system to burn the energetic substances stored in the tissues at a higher and more intense rate.

Physical exercise can also be beneficial to the body by relaxing the mind and the nervous system. In fact, breathlessness and muscular labor will quickly shift attention toward the body. Anxieties, obsessions, tensions, and bad feelings become blurred, at least momentarily, and the physical tensions, spasms, contractions, or blockages they engender disappear. The organs of the body can once more function freely without any disturbance to their activity or malfunctioning due to tensions and blockages of nervous origin.

Whatever physical activity is chosen (walking, biking, tennis, swimming, jogging, etc.), it should be performed according to the individual's physical strengths and capabilities but must last long enough for its effects to reach the deeper regions of the body. It should also take place on a daily basis in order to truly reinforce the benefits of the cure.

OTHER MODALITIES

There are a great many other modalities that can be used as supplements to a whey cure, including hydrotherapy, sauna, massage, and foot reflexology. Each of these techniques will help the body release and eliminate the toxins that are responsible for ill health.

Appendix 1

The Basic Principles of Detoxification Cures

〜

The great efficacy of a whey cure can be fully grasped only when it is placed in the larger context of the detoxification cures used in naturopathic medicine and when one understands the basic principles of this school of medicine.*

In fact, by itself, whey does not directly cure all the diseases and disorders cited as being receptive to its

---

*Much of the material in this appendix has been drawn from my book *The Detox Mono Diet* (Rochester, Vt.: Healing Arts Press, 2006).

active principles. Rather, it works in an indirect manner by positively altering the internal cellular environment, thereby removing the conditions responsible for the hatching and subsistence of the diseases in question. Here, we will consider how this is possible and examine the foundations on which this approach is based.

According to naturopathic medicine, there is an ideal composition of the bodily fluids (blood, lymph, and extracellular and intracellular fluids) in which the cells are immersed; this allows for the optimum functioning of the organs and consequently the body as a whole. Any qualitative modification of these fluids represents a threat to health.

These changes can occur when the internal cellular environment becomes overburdened with substances, such as toxins and poisons, that should not be present in the body or substances, such as uric acid and urea, that should not be present in such large quantities. The other possible cause of these changes is dietary deficiencies—when the body lacks the substances, such as vitamins and minerals, that it requires to maintain the fluids' ideal composition. It is the first problem, the presence of excess amounts of certain substances in the internal environment, that we seek to remedy with detoxification remedies such as the whey cure.

ILLNESS: AN ACCUMULATION OF TOXINS

The concept of illness as a consequence of the presence of undesirable substances in the system is based on observation and can be verified by anybody. Individuals suffering from respiratory ailments blow their noses, cough, and expectorate to rid themselves of the substances that are burdening their alveoli (asthma), their bronchi (bronchitis), their throat (cough), their sinuses (sinusitis), or their nose (the common cold).

The joints of people afflicted with rheumatism and arthritis are inflamed, blocked, and deformed by the presence of grit and crystalline precipitates.

All skin disorders are due to the excretion of either acidic substances by the sudoriferous glands (eczema, skin that is cracked or split) or colloidal substances by the sebaceous glands (acne, boils, greasy skin, sweating, eczema).

Excess food substances in the stomach and intestines can cause indigestion, nausea, vomiting, and diarrhea. When these substances are irritating or fermenting and putrefying, they cause inflammation of the mucous membranes (gastritis, enteritis, colitis) and the production of gas (flatulence, bloating).

The entire gamut of cardiovascular diseases, to which 37 percent of all U.S. deaths are attributed,* is due to the presence of excess substances such as cholesterol and fatty acids that thicken the blood, become deposited on the vessels (arteriosclerosis), inflame the walls (phlebitis, arteritis), deform them (varicose veins), and clog them (heart attack, stroke, embolisms).

In kidney diseases, the guilty substances are protein wastes; in obesity, fats; in cancer, carcinogenic substances; in allergies, allergens; and in stomach ulcers, acids.

THE PROFOUND NATURE OF DISEASE

Our ancient ancestors already knew, and it remains valid today, that the majority of illness is caused by the presence of undesirable substances in the body. These substances have been known by a wide variety of names over the course of history. Today they are generally designated as toxins. These include the cholesterol and fatty acids that are the origin of all the cardiovascular diseases; the acids and crystals that inflame, block, and deform the joints

---

*According to the American Heart Association (www.americanheart.org/presenter.jhtml?identifier=4478)

of those who suffer from rheumatism and arthritis; the colloidal wastes that cause congestion in the respiratory tract, leading to infection and catarrh; the uric acid that causes gout; the salt that retains water; and the sugar that is the root cause of diabetic disorders.

In the present day we must also include in the list of undesirable substances all the food additives (colorings, preservatives), agriculture and gardening products (herbicides, fungicides, insecticides), drugs given to livestock (hormones, antibiotics, vaccines), medications we ourselves take (sedatives, sleeping pills, antibiotics), as well as the large number of poisons stemming from the pollution of our air, water, and earth.

The great doctors of all eras have underscored the fundamental role played by intoxication (in the clinical sense of poisoning). Hippocrates, the father of medicine, wrote: "The nature of all illness is the same. . . . When the contaminated humor is abundant, it will take hold and cast into sickness all that is healthy. The entire body is attacked and thrown out of order."

Thomas Sydenham, a great English doctor of the seventeenth century, summed up the disease process magnificently when he said: "A disease, however much its cause may be adverse to the human body, is nothing more than an effort of Nature, who strives with might and main to restore the health of the patient by the elimination of the morbific [disease-causing] humor."

Closer to our time, the French doctor Paul Carton, dubbed the "Hippocrates of the twentieth century," said in confirmation of the above sentiment: "Disease is in reality only the translation of an inner effort to neutralize and clean out toxins, which the body performs for preservation and regeneration."

Rudolf Steiner, who in the early twentieth century founded anthroposophical medicine, an approach that integrates the physical and spiritual components of the individual, also observed that the origin of internal disorders stems from the fact "that undesirable substances are dissolving into our liquid being."

Whatever the terminology employed in whatever era, disease has always been recognized as being caused by a build-up of substances that clog the body.

THE EXCRETORY ORGANS:
THE EXIT DOORS FOR TOXINS

The body is equipped with five organs for confronting rising levels of toxins: the liver, intestines, kidneys, skin, and lungs. These excretory organs filter wastes out of the blood and the lymph and expel them from the body.

The liver is incontestably the most important of these five organs because not only does it filter and eliminate wastes like the others, it is also capable (if in good health and functioning sufficiently) of neutralizing numerous toxic and carcinogenic substances. The wastes filtered by the liver are eliminated in the bile. Good production and flow of bile is therefore not only a guarantee for good digestion, it also ensures good detoxification.

Because of their combined length (approximately 7 meters or 23 feet) and their diameter (ranging from 3 to 8 centimeters), the intestines also play a fundamental role in waste elimination. In fact, the amount of substances that can stagnate, putrefy, or ferment within them is enormous, and largely contributes to the autointoxication (self-poisoning) of the body.

The kidneys eliminate the wastes filtered out of the blood by diluting them in the urine, insofar as the kidneys are functioning properly. Any reduction in the quantity of urine or its concentration of wastes will engender an accumulation of toxins in the body, and this will generally cause health problems.

The skin constitutes a double exit door as it expels crystalloidal and acid wastes with sweat (through the sudoriferous glands) and colloidal wastes and fats with the sebum (through the sebaceous glands).

The lungs and respiratory tract are primarily an eliminatory path for gaseous wastes, but because of overeating and pollution, they will often expel solid wastes (mucus, spit, and so forth).

TO HEAL MEANS TO DETOXIFY

The solution to the congestion of the body by toxins is detoxification. Nature reveals the path we should follow here. When confronted by excessive wastes, the body reacts: it burns them by fever or seeks to eliminate them through the excretory organs. We can see the wastes leaving the body by way of the skin (acne, eczema), the respiratory tract (bronchitis, colds, sinusitis), the urinary tract (polyuria, acidic urine, grit), the digestive tract (vomiting, diarrhea), the uterus (white discharges), and the eyes (crust or discharge in the eyes on waking, conjunctivitis caused by excess acid in the tears).

If the body is unable to expel all of the wastes via its normal exit channels, the body will create new ones for itself. These may be in the form of varicose ulcers, leaking wounds that will not scar over, or spontaneous hemorrhaging (hemorrhoids, bloody noses, heavy menstruation).

Animals also heal themselves through detoxification. Wolves who are bitten by poisonous snakes cure themselves by purging the toxins with the help of medicinal plants that they would not otherwise eat. When dogs and cats are sick, they will eat grass, which, depending on the amount ingested, can trigger expectoration, diuresis, and vomiting.

THERAPEUTIC DRAINING

"All diseases are resolved either by the mouth, the bowels, the bladder, or some such organ. Sweat is a common form of resolution in all these cases," writes Hippocrates. If illness is caused by autointoxication, it is logical that only detoxification can deal with it successfully. Draining is the method that is used to achieve this cleansing.

Draining consists of stimulating the excretory organs, which are used by the body to filter blood and eliminate toxins. The means that effect this stimulation are varied. They may include using medicinal plants, ingesting fluids and foods that have detoxifying properties (such as whey, for example), adhering to diets, stimulating reflex zones, receiving massages, cleansing the intestines with enemas, and using hydrotherapy.

The excretory organs are the essential pathways

through which this draining is achieved. In draining cures, therapeutic efforts are directed at these organ systems to restore normal elimination and even increase elimination for a period to make up for the buildup of wastes in the body.

First, the individual excretory organ, stimulated by one or more drainers, will cleanse itself of the wastes that lie stagnant in its tissues and clog its "filter." Once it has been cleansed, the organ will regain its ability to filter blood properly. The blood, in turn, irrigates deep tissues, ridding them of accumulated toxins by transporting wastes to the various excretory organs.

Draining is thus characterized by the increased waste elimination performed by excretory organs. This increased elimination will be apparent to the individual taking the cure: The intestines will expel more matter, or evacuation will occur more regularly. Urine, now loaded with wastes, will take on a darker color and will increase in volume. The skin will sweat more copiously, and the respiratory tract will free itself of colloidal wastes through increased coughing and catarrh.

This visible elimination of wastes reduces the amount of toxins that are held in the tissues. With this cleansing of the internal cellular environment comes improvement of the body's overall health and the gradual disappearance of symptoms of illness. The extent of the healing possible obviously depends on the amount of damage that these wastes have already caused in the organs, as well as on these organs' capacity to regenerate.

If draining toxins is not the logical response to the true nature of illnesses, how do we explain that a single therapy—the general draining of toxins—can dispel all health problems for the same patient, despite the vast differences that might characterize the disorders?

A multitude of patients, after running from one specialist to the next to treat various disorders, have found themselves cured of *all* conditions by a single causal treatment—detoxification with therapeutic drainers.

THE IMPORTANCE OF MAINTAINING GOOD EXCRETORY FUNCTION

The excretory organs serve as the obligatory exit doors for toxins. The following figures illustrate the importance of these organs and the consequences that may result when any of them loses function.

The kidneys should eliminate 25–30 grams of urea over a twenty-four-hour period. If they eliminate only 20 grams, this represents retention of at least 5 grams per day, or 150 grams (⅓ pound) per month! These

〜

150 grams of urea will clog the tissues and overburden the internal cellular environment. The same is true for salt. If the kidneys eliminate 12 grams of salt in twenty-four hours, instead of the entire 15 or more grams that are typically absorbed from food, this means 3 grams each day are retained, equaling 90 grams (⅕ pound) per month!

To be sure, these elimination figures are not precise, as wastes can be expelled through more than one exit. Nevertheless, substantial amounts of wastes do accumulate in the tissues, as can be seen during dialysis.

During one twenty-four-hour period of blood dialysis —in which all blood is extracted from the arteries and passed through a filter that removes urea before the blood is reintroduced through a vein—an amount of 300–400 grams of urea can be collected, whereas the presence of only a few grams (2 grams per liter of blood) is considered fatal. These 300–400 grams of urea are obviously not stored in the bloodstream (our bodies contain only around 5 liters of blood, so this amount would clearly be fatal); but, because the excretory organs are unable to eliminate all of the wastes, they are pushed deeper into the tissues where they contribute to congestion of the internal environment.

RECOGNIZING GOOD EXCRETORY FUNCTION

The criteria for good excretory function are as follows: the intestines should empty once a day; the stools should be well formed but not hard, and they should not have a foul odor. The speed at which food travels through the intestines is also important. Food should leave the body within twenty-four to thirty-six hours after it is consumed. Hard, dry stools that are difficult to expel and are evacuated only every two to three days or more are a sign of autointoxication in the intestines, characterized by poor elimination.

The kidneys eliminate approximately 1.3 liters of urine each day. Urine should contain certain wastes that are detectable only through analysis, but which give urine its typical color and odor. Consequently, urine that is too clear, has no color or odor, or is excreted too infrequently (meaning only two or three urinations a day) indicates insufficient kidney function. Urine that is highly charged with wastes testifies to strong eliminatory capacity, but also reveals a high level of contamination.

The skin eliminates wastes through the sudoriferous glands in the form of a liquid (sweat) and through the sebaceous glands as a greasy coating (sebum). Healthy skin perspires over its entire surface and maintains its suppleness thanks to secretions of sebum. The absence of perspiration, acne, and the various forms of eczema can indicate that the skin is sealed and the wastes it should be eliminating are stagnating below the surface.

The respiratory tract (lungs, bronchi, nasopharynx, sinuses) provides paths of elimination for gaseous wastes (CO_2). It should not be obstructed by solid or fluid wastes (phlegm, mucus, colloidal wastes). Congestion is a sign that the body as a whole has accumulated too many toxins and is trying to expel some of them through the respiratory tract. Except for a few waste products present when rising in the morning, the nose should always be clear and free of congestion.

THE DRAINERS

Drainers are the products used to stimulate the excretory organs to perform their filtering and elimination tasks. Drainers, in addition to their eliminatory effect, also regulate and reeducate the excretory organs to restore optimum function. Drainers consist of simple foods as well as medicinal plants that have specific properties that encourage the work of the excretory organs. Some of the most effective drainers for each of the excretory organs are listed here.

HEPATIC DRAINERS

- Artichoke, dandelion, black radish, carrot, cabbage
- Infusions, drops, or tablets of common centaury *(Centaurium minus)*, rosemary, chicory, dandelion, black radish, boldo, curcuma
- Olive oil: Take 1–2 tablespoons in the morning on an empty stomach. This treatment should be followed for fifteen days.

INTESTINAL DRAINERS

- Wheat bran
- Flax seeds, psyllium, agar-agar powder
- Prunes, figs
- Infusions, drops, or tablets of alder buckthorn, cassia, mallow, licorice, polypody
- Whey

RENAL DRAINERS

- Artichoke, asparagus, pumpkin, watercress, green beans, cabbage, celery, onion, turnip, pear
- Infusion, drops, or tablets of linden sapwood, birch, bearberry leaves, cherry stem, horsetail, couch grass, dandelion, juniper, nettle, onion, leeks
- Drinking lots of fluids: water with low mineral content, fruit and vegetable juices, whey, herbal teas

PULMONARY DRAINERS

- Juice, infusions, tablets, or essential oils of
  eucalyptus, oregano, plantain, licorice, coltsfoot,
  Iceland moss, thyme

CUTANEOUS DRAINERS

- Juice, infusions, drops, or tablets of burdock,
  borage, chamomile, wild pansy, elder, lime
  blossom
- Hot baths, saunas, warm compresses
- Massage with gentle essential oils like lavender or
  geranium

As we have seen, whey is an intestinal drainer as well
as a renal drainer, and it has an indirect effect upon the
liver. Whey acts on three of the five excretory organs—
hence its great effectiveness in detoxifying the body.

THE PRACTICE OF DRAINING CURES

Two factors must be taken into consideration with draining cures: their intensity and duration.

The efficacy of the draining will depend on its intensity. Therefore, determining the correct dosage is key: if
it's too low, the excretory organ will not receive enough

stimulation and no results will be obtained; if the dose is set too high, the body will exhaust itself and the excretory organs themselves can become damaged from the flood of toxins. The optimum dose, one that sits somewhere between these two extremes, will be different for each individual body. Unfortunately there are no mathematical formulas for determining the correct dosage. Each individual must start with a small dose and gradually increase the amount, while monitoring the body's reactions, to determine the appropriate dosage. Beginning with a large dose can cause imbalances and puts the body at risk for exhaustion. In addition to the general health threat this poses, it also makes it difficult to determine the body's true reaction to the drainer.

The duration of the draining also plays a fundamental role in the success of the treatment. The cleansing engendered by the draining is a physiological process. The body is not capable of emptying itself of all its toxins at once. To the contrary, toxins are extracted from the blood and tissues little by little. For a detoxification cure to be effective, drainers should be used regularly for at least two weeks, preferably for a duration of one to two months. Cures can be repeated several times during the year as needed, so long as the body is given a month-long rest in between treatments.

∽

All of the excretory organs should not necessarily be stimulated at the same time. When draining is practiced for the first time, it is preferable to stimulate only one organ at a time to avoid dispersing the body's strength. In this case, begin with the organ that is the most deficient: the intestines in cases of constipation, the kidneys in cases of edema, and so on.

Another option is to stimulate the excretory organs in order of their importance: liver, intestines, kidneys, skin, and lungs. This progression is even more prudent for the individual who is suffering from a great degree of poisoning (someone who eats a lot of meat or has been overmedicated) or whose energy reserves and strength are restricted (the elderly or those who have been severely ill). Once the excretory organs have been retrained, the draining cures can target all the eliminatory organs at the same time. The organs will be more responsive to detoxification efforts and will eliminate wastes more efficiently, leading to better overall health.

Appendix 2

Nutritional Analysis of Powdered Whey

∽

AVERAGE NUTRITIONAL COMPOSITION
PER 100 GRAMS

Lactose	75 g
Protein	12 g
Minerals	8 g
Water	4 g
Lipids	1 g

Nutritional Analysis of Powdered Whey

MINERAL COMPOSITION PER 100 GRAMS*

Potassium	2.0 g
Calcium	0.7 g
Magnesium	0.1 g
Phosphorus	0.8 g
Sodium	0.9 g
Chlorine	1.6 g

*Those minerals present in whey in very low quantities have been excluded from this table.

VITAMIN COMPOSITION PER 100 GRAMS

Vitamin A	0.015 mg
Vitamin B_1	0.490 mg
Vitamin B_2	2,500 mg
Vitamin B_3	0.800 mg
Vitamin C	1000 mg

Resources

POWDERED WHEY

Powdered whey is widely available, with many companies offering their own brands. Companies such as **Biosana** (www.biosana.ch/e/company.html) and **Next Proteins' Designer Whey** (www.designerwhey.com) offer a variety of flavors. For those following a whey cure, it is best to use natural pure whey powder and avoid those products that have additional supplements and flavors (some of which are artificial). Other companies manufacturing or distributing whey powder are ISS Research, Prolab Nutrition, Swanson Premium Brand, EAS, GNC, Twinlab, and Country Life.

SPA WHEY CURES

It is still possible to take the old-fashioned whey cure in Europe. Many spas in the United States and Europe offer whey baths as part of their treatments, but not the whey cure. The principal location still remains the Appenzell region of Switzerland, which is about one hour's travel time by car or train from Zurich. At least two of the many spas in this region offer traditional whey cures; their contact information is listed here.

Kurhaus Bad Gonten
9108 Gotenbad—Appenzell
Switzerland
Telephone: 41 (0) 71 794 11 24
Fax: 41 (0) 71 794 16 60
www.badgonten.ch
info@badgonten.ch

Hotel Hof Weissbad
9057 Weissbad—Appenzell
Switzerland
Telephone: 41 (0) 71 798 80 80
Fax: 41 (0) 71 798 80 90
www.hofweissbad.ch
hotel@hofweissbad.ch

Resources

AUTHOR'S WEB SITE

www.christophervasey.ch
The author presents his different books and provides for each of them the table of contents and a general introduction to the subject of the book. The Web site also contains biographical information, a calendar of events, and links to related sites.

Index

Index

Index

joint diseases, 41

kidneys
  drainers for, 76
  medicinal plants and, 56
  toxin elimination and,
    29–31, 67–68, 72–73,
    74
  whey and, 41
kidney stones, 42, 57

L+ lactic acid, 15–16
lactic acid, 12, 14–16, 24
lactose, 8–9, 11–14, 16,
  25–26
lactose intolerance, 52
laxatives, 12, 24–25
legs, 28
lipids, 8, 9, 16
liquid whey, 8–9, 45
liver, 26–28, 27, 42, 56, 67–68,
  76
lungs, 67–69, 75
lymph, 32
lymphatic stasis, 29

magnesium, 12, 20
manufacturers, of whey, 46
massage, 61
meat, 18
medications, 66
medicinal plants, 55–57
memory loss, 21
milk, 7–8, 18
minerals, 19–21, 31

mono diets, 50–51
mucous membranes, 14, 27–28

naturopathy, 62–63
nerve impulses, 19, 20
nettles, 56–57
nutritional content, of whey
  caloric intake, 16–17
  lactic acid, 14–16
  lactose, 11–14
  lipids, 16
  minerals, 19–21
  of powdered, 80–81
  proteins, 17–19
  vitamins, 21–22
  See also whey

organ congestion, 29
osteoarthritis, 30, 41
osteoporosis, 20
oxidation, 58
oxygenation, 57–60

peristalsis, 12, 24, 38–39
phosphorus, 12, 21
plants, medicinal, 55–57
potassium, 9, 12, 19–20
powdered whey, 6, 9, 46,
  80–81, 82
proteins, 8–9, 17–19
pulmonary drainers, 77
putrefaction, 13–14, 31

raw milk, 7–8
reflexology, 61

BOOKS OF RELATED INTEREST

The Acid–Alkaline Diet for Optimum Health
Restore Your Health by Creating pH Balance in Your Diet
by Christopher Vasey, N.D.

The Detox Mono Diet
The Miracle Grape Cure and Other Cleansing Diets
by Christopher Vasey, N.D.

The Water Prescription
For Health, Vitality, and Rejuvenation
by Christopher Vasey, N.D.

Optimal Digestive Health: A Complete Guide
Edited by Trent W. Nichols, M.D., and Nancy Faass, MSW, MPH

Amino Acids in Therapy
A Guide to the Therapeutic Application of Protein Constituents
by Leon Chaitow, D.O., N.D.

The High Blood Pressure Solution
A Scientifically Proven Program for
Preventing Strokes and Heart Disease
by Richard D. Moore, M.D., Ph.D.

Colloidal Minerals and Trace Elements
How to Restore the Body's Natural Vitality
by Marie-France Muller, M.D., N.D., Ph.D.

The Whole Food Bible
How to Select & Prepare Safe, Healthful Foods
by Chris Kilham

Inner Traditions • Bear & Company
P.O. Box 388
Rochester, VT 05767
1-800-246-8648
www.InnerTraditions.com

Or contact your local bookseller

PLEASE SEND US THIS CARD TO RECEIVE OUR LATEST CATALOG.

Book in which this card was found _____

☐ Check here if you would like to receive our catalog via e-mail.

Name _____ Company _____

Address _____ Phone _____

City _____ State _____ Zip _____ Country _____

E-mail address _____

Please check the following area(s) of interest to you:

☐ Health   ☐ Self-help   ☐ Science/Nature   ☐ Shamanism

☐ Ancient Mysteries   ☐ New Age/Spirituality   ☐ Ethnobotany   ☐ Martial Arts

☐ Spanish Language   ☐ Sexuality/Tantra   ☐ Children   ☐ Teen

Please send a catalog to my friend:

Name _____ Company _____

Address _____ Phone _____

City _____ State _____ Zip _____ Country _____

Order at 1-800-246-8648 • Fax (802) 767-3726

E-mail: customerservice@InnerTraditions.com • Web site: www.InnerTraditions.com

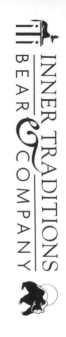

INNER TRADITIONS
BEAR & COMPANY

Inner Traditions • Bear & Company

P.O. Box 388

Rochester, VT 05767-0388

U.S.A.

Affix
Postage
Stamp
Here